Checks & Balances

A Practical Approach to Optimal Health and Wellness

Steve Thompson, MPT

Checks and Balances

Published by:
90-Minute Books
302 Martinique Drive
Winter Haven, FL 33884
www.90minutebooks.com

Copyright © 2015, Steve Thompson, MPT

Published in the United States of America

ISBN-13: 978- 0692504949
ISBN-10: 069250494X

For more information on 90-Minute Books including finding out how you can publish your own lead generating book, visit www.90minutebook.com or call (863) 318-0464

Here's What's Inside...

September 2015

Most people don't know this, but physical therapy has been around since around World War I. It started, in fact, as a result of all the soldiers coming back injured from the war. It has evolved a lot since then.

During the 1970s, the primary treatment one would receive when going to a physical therapist would be to get hot packs, ultrasounds, and massages. That was pretty much the extent of physical therapy. Maybe you would have received a few exercises to do, but you really didn't get a whole lot out of those visits. In the last decade, there has been a huge growth within our profession and more understanding that what we do is very beneficial and more cost effective than many medical procedures. Due to improved technology, physical therapy is more evidence-based, and overwhelmingly the profession is showing that exercise is one of the most valuable components of long-term correction and outcome from an injury.

In the last 10 to 20 years, there has been a growth in manual therapy and exercise techniques. Now we have a great variety of different ways to approach someone who is in pain. Highly skilled physical therapists can determine what is truly wrong with a patient with greater efficiency and effectiveness. Even with all of the information and technology available to physical therapists and the greater skills that we have, often times, when we get a referral from a doctor—let's say it's a patient with back pain—the most common diagnosis is degenerated disc disease, which really does not tell us much. What people don't realize is that the term degenerative disc disease is related to a natural aging process, but one that can be improved and managed effectively.

Typically, during the first visit I ask them, "First of all, did your doctor explain what's going on with you?" Generally the first response is "No." Then I will ask, "Do you understand what this diagnosis means?" Again, they answer "No." Unfortunately, people are being diagnosed, labeled, and sent to physical therapy but have no idea what is going on with their health. This is where physical therapy shines; we take the time to educate our patients on not only the problem but the root cause as well.

I think the old school physical therapy is of the mindset, "If I give you a fish I feed you for a day" whereas the modern physical therapist is about, "If I teach you how to fish, I feed you for a lifetime." Our job is to keep people out of the healthcare system, to get them healthy and balanced so that they don't need to keep coming back. We educate our clients so they can take personal responsibility for their lives. We help people restore their dysfunctions and movement patterns to ones that can give them the longest and healthiest life.

I hope this book educates you about your approach to wellness and encourages you to add physical therapy to your health and wellness tool kit.

To Your Success!

Steve Thompson, MPT

Checks and Balances

The idea for this book has grown out of my 20 years as a physical therapist and helping people overcome injuries and achieve better health and wellness. I wanted to have a positive effect on the largest number of people in the simplest way possible, beyond what we see in our clinics.

One of my mentors, Tim McGonigle, PT, introduced me to the concept of managing lower back pain by simply considering managing back pain much like managing your checking account balance. What I mean by that is considering that there are activities we do that can aggravate our injuries (spend money) and there are activities that we CAN do to improve our health (deposit money).

If we follow the simple rules of do what is good for you and avoid what is not good for you, we can get ourselves out of pain, improve our health and wellness, and prevent pains from coming back. These are rather simple ideas, but if applied to our everyday lifestyles, they can dramatically affect our lives for the better—or for the worse, if someone chooses to ignore the pains or bad activities.

Now, if you consider your own checking account balance, you always strive to keep money in the bank, right? However, we voluntarily spend money every day and there are expenses that we cannot avoid, both of which involve writing checks that will deplete our account.

In order to prevent our checking account from being overdrawn, we MUST continually put money into the account so we can afford our lifestyles. It is simply a game of debits and credits. Inflow has to be greater than outflow. Basic economics and many financial experts would agree with this.

Unfortunately, many Americans are saddled with debt, habitually spending more than we have in the bank and then taking out loans and credit cards to allow us to keep up with our lifestyle. Sooner or later, we will get to the point where we can't pay our bills and file for bankruptcy. People are not paying attention to the correct philosophy of taking responsibility for their own financial security and end up going into deeper financial debt.

Unfortunately, many are not saving enough to retire and will depend on government assistance, such as Medicare and Social Security, for their retirement. This is creating a crisis for our economy and adding significant stress to our financial markets and ourselves.

The same analogy can be used to analyze and explain the personal health care crises we have now. Over the past 20 years, I have tried to educate my patients that the path to better health and wellness is very similar to our checking account balances. If we do activities that are costly to our bodies, our health, and our well-being and at the same time don't do enough to be restorative and healthy, we will reach a point where our body's checking account balance will dip below '0' and we will be in debt. Basically, we will be writing checks our bodies can't cash and, eventually, something breaks. Once we dip below zero, we experience pain. The greater in 'debt' we are to our bodies, the more pain we feel, the poorer our health becomes, the more stressed we feel, and in general, the sicker we get.

For example, if we think about this concept in terms of lower back pain, then managing back pain can become easier and we can actually prevent back pain from occurring or manage it more effectively when we do have pain. There are activities we do that place significant strain on our lower backs, such as sitting and driving, bending and lifting with poor body mechanics, living a sedentary life and getting weaker core musculature and extremities. These are all withdrawals on our health accounts. Yet we are expecting that our back will be strong and healthy when we need it.

These negative activities and mechanical stresses are similar to writing big checks when we have plenty of money in our 'bank' (i.e., when we are younger and more resilient) and we don't see the effect of these withdrawals. Unfortunately, at some point, we will exceed our zero balance level, falling into "debt", and then pain will strike. I often tell my patients that they essentially have a trust fund when they are born that has a lot of money in the fund but we do not know exactly how much is in that account. Therefore, we carelessly spend money (do bad activities for ourselves) and at some point suffer from that behavior when we 'overdraw our account' and we are now in pain.

Another way to think about how the account balance relates to our backs is that when we are born, we have a healthy back that allow us to do many activities. We only have so many 'free passes' of getting by with bad bends and lifts. Once you use the last 'freebie', the next lift or bend could be very painful, even if that bend is simply picking up a pencil or sock off the floor.

The easy part about our actual financial checking account is that we can always know where we stand in relation to our balance just by going online with our bank. When we are in the positive, we can write checks and then check to make sure it clears. For our bodies, when we are in the positive, unfortunately we don't know how much money we have in the bank at any time so we just spend recklessly and carelessly by bending and lifting poorly until pain strikes, and then we want an immediate solution to get out of pain.

When we overdraw our financial checking account, again, we can check our account levels with the bank and find out how much we have to deposit to get back in the black. For our bodies, we also can tell how much we are in 'debt' by the level of pain. If we have a low level, chronic pain, we are probably only slightly below the zero balance level and we can do small positive activities, or deposits, to get back in the "black". However, over time, we get numb to the chronic pains and it becomes more constant. Thus, our negative account levels get more negative and it will take bigger and bigger deposits (or positive efforts) to get back in the black. When we do something and suffer extreme pain, we have just written a HUGE check that will take us way into the negative balance levels and it will take a lot to get back out of pain.

We can apply this to a bigger picture that looks very similar to the current national health care crisis that is looming. We do not take care of ourselves well; in fact, we take better care of our houses, cars, pets, material things and others better than we do ourselves! Our lifestyle is one of constantly living in a state of health debt, hoping some new costly technology will be our savior or we rely on Obamacare and the insurance company to cover our healthcare needs. Then, as we get older, we accumulate diseases and health problems, creating a costly, unmanageable health care system that drives us into deeper and deeper debt. This is not a good long-term strategy.

This concept does not have to relate solely to back pain. We can apply the same principles of managing our checking account balances to stress, work, relationships, investments, wellness, sleep, diet, and overall well-being. By actively engaging in more positive and healthy activities and avoiding dangerous and unhealthy ones, we can keep our accounts balanced, so to speak. By taking responsibility for our health, not just someone else's, we can live happier and healthier lives.

I wrote this book to be a source of education and enlightenment for our society. We need to step up our game, stay educated, take care of ourselves first, and take responsibility for ourselves and our well-being. I want this book to open the eyes of our nation to the concept that healthcare is not about being reliant on someone else to take care of our situation and place in life. Healthcare is about self-control; we have the control to manage our health, and health care providers are there to help guide us when we need help.

Why More People Don't Have Optimum Health and Wellness

Our society is riddled with debt-laden, credit-burdened people living outside of their means, living in stressed lives every day wondering where to get the money to pay their bills, asking the government for bail outs and handouts because we are entitled to live the way we choose to live. They are not taking responsibility for their own lives and situations, demanding that someone else take care of them, such as insurance companies and government assistance.

With respect to health, the analogy is very much the same—the vast majority of us suffer from pain every day. In fact, at some point in their lives, 90% of the population will suffer from lower back pain that can last six to eight weeks at a minimum.

We are more obese, more stressed, have more autoimmune disorders, have more allergies, are more sedentary, and generally unhealthier than we have ever been before in our history. Americans are overwhelmed with information, stress, indecision, relationship problems, health problems, and financial problems to the point where we are stuck, not moving forward to a better place in life. We point our fingers outward for the solution when we should simply look in the mirror as the source of a better way.

At the same time, we are living longer than ever before, which basically means that we will suffer for longer periods of time in our lives unless we do something about our own state of health and wellness. This is all occurring when we have some of the most cutting-edge technology and have more information at our fingertips than ever before, with some of the best-trained health providers available to us. People suffer from orthopedic injuries on a daily basis and the numbers are growing exponentially. Our young athletes are suffering more sports-related injuries than ever before, and yet we are not doing anything to correct this problem. Left unmanaged, these issues will have the potential to crush our society under a debt from which we cannot recover.

If people simply look at their lives and analyze where they are now, where they want to be, and then figure out what obstacles are contributing to the condition they are in, they can easily apply the strategy of "money in, money out" to get into a better state of health and wellness.

From there, people could discover for themselves what causes them to suffer from stress, pain, anxiety, poor health, poor diet, and obesity. They can then look at what makes them feel better and live better—what reduces pain, stress, injury, and weight gain—and engage in those things that are good for them in greater quantity and less of what is bad for them (or eliminate what is bad for them). They can now start on a path toward a happier, healthier (body-wise and economically) lives and we can begin to grow and reduce the burdens on our society versus continuing the way we are currently living and creating greater demands on our already stressed government and economy.

Were people to apply this easy formula of reducing their health debits and always look to make 'deposits' into their own accounts, they would become dramatically more productive, happier, and more prosperous (health and money-wise).

We would also reduce the burdens on the health care system, and I would probably put myself out of a job as a physical therapist. If that did happen, what a great world this would be. I do believe that if our world was healthier, then physical therapists would become more like health coaches rather than healthcare providers.

If people choose to ignore this simple solution, we are headed for a nation of people with catastrophic health conditions and a crumbling state of healthcare. We will depend on others for our survival, which will end up costing our system significantly more money than it costs today. Technology is already helping us to live longer, and there are predictions that with technology we will be able to live for significantly longer than the current predicted lifespan. However, if we continue to live in a debt-driven way, we will suffer through most of those hundreds of years.

Optimum health and wellness begins when you look in the mirror and hold yourself accountable for you FIRST. Only then will we begin to gain more control, more power, achieve better health, have more enjoyment, live with less pain, suffer fewer injuries, get more out of life, have less stress, and so many more benefits that we are not even aware of yet! Wouldn't it be a great place if we achieved this? Taking control of any situation is empowering, and this can lead to greater personal and professional growth and more security in life and a fantastic future.

The Eight Steps to Attaining Optimum Health and Wellness

If you break it down – getting healthy is actually pretty simple. It may not be easy, but IT IS SIMPLE. By working through these eight steps, anyone can tackle any challenge or negative state they are in and turn their lives around for the positive. It will take work, but it can be done.

1. GET CLARITY ON WHERE YOU ARE NOW AND WHAT YOU WANT TO CHANGE

We must start with where we are in life to determine where we want to go. This is a very important first step, and we must be COMPLETELY honest and truthful with ourselves about this step.

For example, someone may review their life and notice that they do not have enough money, are not saving any money, have occasional to frequent back pain, neck tightness, obesity, a failing marriage or relationship, are unsatisfied with their job, or whatever it is that is real to them. At this point, we have to be honest with ourselves and write down where we are and be careful not be judgmental or critical of where we are. It is very easy to allow our inner critics to have a field day at this stage and to derail any further progress.

Next, we need to decide what it is we want—better health, less stress, lose weight, less pain, be able to drive to and from work and sit at the desk without pain, or whatever is real to us. This is a foundational development step. Without this clarity, you will have a tough time moving forward.

This step has to be objective and free from emotion. The reader may want to consult a specialist to help determine where they are now and where they could be; for example, go see your doctor and get a health checkup and find out where you are and where you should be if you were healthy. You may want to seek the advice of physical therapists to determine what is weak and what is tight and out of balance. Find all of the professionals you can to help you determine objectively where you are now and what you could do in the future if you committed to this process.

Make your own personal goals and ideal conditions. Again, this step is not easy, but it is critical to moving forward. List each of the areas of your life that you want to improve on and list an end result you want to achieve. Be specific and detailed.

2. NOTE WHERE THE 'MONEY' IS FLOWING OUTWARD

Let's take back pain again as an example. One thing you could do is spend a little time analyzing everything that makes your back pain worse. Log it and measure the time it takes the pain to get worse. Here you begin to make a list of what 'checks' you are writing and how much it costs you, and you will have the first raw materials to reduce your pain.

You can apply this process to every area of your life that you want to change. For money, look at what you are spending and identify the necessary items that you have to pay in order to live. For stress, pay attention to how you feel throughout the day. When a headache or neck ache arises, note specifically what activity you are doing or maybe the person with whom you are interacting at that time. For diet, pay attention to what you eat, even log it, and then note how you feel and what symptoms you experience. In a relationship, note how you feel with your partner, your friends, your boss, your co-workers, and who makes your feel bad and what it is about that situation that contributes to the condition. For exercise, note how you feel after a workout. In particular, did you have any abnormal pains? Log it all.

Here you are identifying all of the 'checks and outflows' in your life's account. Be as specific as possible. When we chart activities specifically measuring how much it costs, how long it takes to worsen, etc., we can create a goal to strive for.

3. NOTE WHAT BRINGS MONEY INTO YOUR ACCOUNT

Now, for the back pain person, determine what you do that lessens your pain, such as walking, standing, exercise, lying down, changing positions, etc., and how long it takes to do these activities to reduce the back pain. For the other areas of your life, repeat this process.

For stress and mental health, note what gives you energy and makes you feel good, happy, and fulfilled. For diet, what foods do you eat that give you energy and make you feel satiated. For exercise, what is the activity and what variables are part of that exercise that make you feel good—is it indoors or outdoors, alone or in a group, more cardio-based or strength-based? Here you are identifying the deposits and inflows of your life's account. From here, we now have the sources of getting to a better state and we know how much 'money in' we have to put into our accounts to feel better.

4. MAKE THE COMMITMENT TO BRING MORE 'MONEY' INTO YOUR ACCOUNT THAN WHAT GOES OUT

We all love games. Make this process fun and energizing. If you approach with drudgery, you will not be successful. Remember, you are on the road to improving your lifestyle and your future, which should be exciting and energizing!

Now that you have established where you are and where you want to go and have the specifics of what is working for you and what is not, you have the raw ingredients for building a better life. To gain confidence and accomplish anything in life, we must start with a full commitment to the process of change. In our clinics, the patients who don't do well are often the ones who do not fully commit to getting better. That sounds strange, doesn't it? What I mean by this is that people are coming to physical therapy to get better but many people are truly not committed to getting better. But much like what I have described, where people tend to put their cars, houses, pets, and others ahead of themselves, the same ones do not fully commit to healing. They are the ones who don't do their home exercises, don't pay attention to their own progress, often cancel because of hair and nail appointments, and often get frustrated with physical therapy that they are not further along than they wanted to be. Then they blame the process or physical therapy instead of taking responsibility for their own success.

Commitment is everything. As Dan Sullivan, the founder of Strategic Coach, says, if you give a half commitment to anything, you will get half results and you will spend more time suffering through the process of improvement and end up being disappointed in the progress or lack thereof. Go into this with a full commitment and WANTING the desired changes, not NEEDING improvement. You never want to approach your commitment with 'I

NEED to make a change' as it will result in a weak commitment, but rather approach it with I WANT to make a change.

For example, the most difficult clients to work with are those who have dealt with chronic low back pain because it is just not bad enough and they don't WANT to put the time and effort in to get better. Remember the account balance is just under zero when it is bad but the person is not committed enough to do something about it. The most motivated patients are those that have the greatest need to improve, such as someone who has injured their hand and dominant arm.

5. START SIMPLE AND THEN GO BIG

Many people who want to make changes and are committed to getting better will experience failure if they try to do too many things at once right out of the gate. Also, make sure that you are specific about where you are and where you want to go because our brains will work better when there are specific objective measures to reach. With the list that you've created, start by committing to one thing and one thing only. This will allow you to focus your attention and intentions on improving that area. Once you experience the success of achieving that task, then use that momentum to apply it to other areas on your list.

Intention is a very important concept to understand. Intention is the driver of all things. In order to do something in life, you must INTEND to do it. If you really don't care about improving, you will not improve. If you don't intend to change something, you will never change. Remember the chronic low back pain patient, the chronically stressed person, the person whose diet is 'not that bad'? Deep down, they really do not intend to get better and thus they don't. There will be a compounding effect to daily wear and tear, meaning it will get worse if you don't commit.

6. MEASURE AND REPORT YOUR IMPROVEMENTS

Pearson's Law states, "That which is measured improves. That which is measured and reported improves dramatically." This law is so true. When you are beginning this quest for improvement, make sure you share it with someone. I don't mean on Facebook or Twitter; share it with someone special, a co-worker, a team, or a great friend. Just by measuring your progress, you will hold yourself accountable, and this will raise your intentions to improve and the results will follow. Trying to make the changes in your life objective and measurable allows you to track your improvements for yourself, which will guarantee that you will improve.

However, if you want exponential improvements, enlist someone who you feel comfortable with and will support you on your quest, and share it with them on a regular basis and ask that they keep you accountable. When you have successes, report them to your partner to celebrate. Celebrate any win, big or small.

For example, if back pain is your main issue, when you can sit at your desk and work for half of a day without pain, when you started at 15 minutes, celebrate that! You have made exceptional improvements. The reason I say don't report it on Facebook and Twitter is that as you improve yourself and you broadcast that to the world is that

Facebooking or Tweeting your goal is a weak commitment because who will hold you accountable. Also, unfortunately, there are many people who are not like you and are not in a positive mindset or growth mindset and will try to tear you down and devalue your progress. Find those with a similar mindset and you will guarantee your results.

Some say who you are in five to 10 years depends on the books you read and the people with whom you associate. Associate with positive people and those who you want to be like, and you will become like them. Hang around those who contribute to the bad habits and poor conditions of your health, and you will set yourself up for failure.

For example, if you want to get in shape, feel better, and get stronger, then hanging around people who go to the gym, are outdoors a lot, and generally look after themselves will help you achieve your goals. If you hang around people who drink at the bars every night, don't know what a gym is, and keep pulling you into those environments, you will fail, guaranteed.

7. REALIZE THAT YOUR GOAL IS POSSIBLE AND ACHIEVABLE

If you make out your list of where you are and what you want to accomplish and then keep your inner critic out of the discussion, you will succeed. If you have lower back pain, you must believe that your goal is possible and that you can live a life without lower back pain as long as you address it, take responsibility for the process, and recruit as many people as needed to help you get to that point.

If you allow your inner critic to judge your goals, you will tell yourself that you will not achieve it and you will find yourself justifying why your path was not successful. Again, using the lower back pain example, patients who start out in physical therapy to improve their lower back pain but are not committed and listen to the naysayers who tell them that it will not work will most likely not do their exercises, will not progress, and their pain will not improve.

These are the patients who often say to us, "See! I told you that I would not get better and that I am always going to have lower back pain!" However, if you surround yourself with those who truly support you and help you move forward and give you the encouragement to succeed, you will.

8. EVEN IF MONEY IS NOT YOUR STRONG SUIT OR SOMETHING YOU UNDERSTAND WELL, THIS CONCEPT WILL WORK

You don't have to be a banker or financial advisor to understand this theory of "Checks and Balances – Money In versus Money Out" as the key to optimal health and wellness. Simply understand that the more positive activities you do versus negative activities you do, you will end up better than before. The saying of 'two steps forward and one step back' still gets you one step forward.

Realize that even though you do something that may cause you more pain or stress or you feel worse after a meal, you do have the ability to make it better. It may take more effort to get back in the positive zone, but you will get there. For example, if you just drove six to eight hours without stopping and now you are suffering from intense lower back pain that threatens to destroy your fun family vacation, you can rectify the situation by doing many of the things that put money back in your back account right away. In this case you could use ice, walk a bit, do the proper exercises and stretch to help put money back in your 'bank'.

Also, based on what happened on the drive down, you now have the ability to make a plan for the return trip home: take frequent stops, get someone else to drive so you can recline, use ice while you drive, and so on.

The Checks and Balances Solution Works for Many Types of People

Over the years, many patients have applied the principles of relating their activities as their checking account balance, as debits and credits, and have successfully eliminated their lower back pain. Nearly everyone who is still applying the principles is pain free still.

For example, with one patient, Mary, whose name is changed, we applied this concept to not only her lower back pain, but also a stressful situation at home with her spouse, with taking care of an abusive elderly parent, and an in-law whom she was taking care of, as they were elderly and dealing with health issues.

Mary had been suffering from many years of emotional abuse from many sources and did not have any tools to use in these situations. When I gave her this analogy, it immediately made sense to her and she began to implement the strategies. She has turned her life around where she is now in control of her parent and in-law situations. She is able to deflect the abusive nature of the relationship and empower herself, and she has more control over her life. She also does not have lower back pain anymore.

I will share my story to help illustrate my point. Prior to 2002, I was in my late 20s and heading into my early 30s. Like many people that age, I felt like I could do whatever I wanted. I was an athlete when I was younger, and I would play tons of golf with my brother and my dad. We would play five rounds of golf in a weekend, which probably wasn't the smartest thing to do.

Around Memorial Day of 2002, I had come back from a weekend of golf. We played five rounds in South Carolina, and then I hopped on a plane, flew home, and started to notice that week that I was having a little bit of back pain. It progressively got more and more uncomfortable until a week later, I woke up and I couldn't stand up. I couldn't stand up for more than about a minute and a half before I had a searing pain going down my right leg as if someone was clenching a vice around my calf. The only thing that gave me relief was to lie on the ground.

I approached my situation using the "checks and balances" philosophy by getting up and moving around for as long as I could before I started to feel the pain again. Then I would do activities that helped relieve the pain, whether that was lying down, icing, stretching, anything and everything that felt good.

I did have to have an injection in the beginning to try to decrease the inflammation. But what I did every day is walk the same path over and over again, trying to see how far I could get. Maybe the first day I was only able to go a quarter mile and then I would turn around and walk home. If my symptoms started to get worse, it was time to go home. I kept following this path each time, trying to do positive things for my back, doing the exercises my physical therapist gave me, and continually doing good activities while minimizing the bad activities.

In the end, I was able to overcome this with no surgery. My back hasn't really bugged me, and now it's been 13 years since, but I know that I am just as susceptible as everybody else is. If I sit too much, if I play too many rounds of golf, I'll feel a little bit of pain. So I know what my limits are now. If I do my exercises every single day, stay healthy, walk, and keep my weight in control, then I don't have any back pain issues. And it's now been 13 years and I'm still going strong!

The Types of Injuries a Physical Therapist Can Help With

Physical therapists are probably one of the most under appreciated healthcare professionals in handling musculoskeletal injuries. Unfortunately, a lot of doctors don't yet see the value in physical therapy, especially primary care physicians. Most of the time when people go to their doctor for lower back pain or something of that sort, that primary care physician does not always know what to do with them. Their first course is usually to give them some medication. I wish that people would realize that if they are having joint pain or a physical muscular skeletal ailment, they should come to us first. We are probably the best ones to evaluate and direct the best course of action. It may be that they need to be referred to a physician, but many times, we can handle things on a much more cost-effective basis for them versus going to the primary care physician, getting an MRI, getting an X-ray, and then finally coming to us. We can handle a majority, if not all, musculoskeletal injuries, but we are also capable of saying, "This is out of our realm," and refer to the physician. They are better off starting with us versus the other way around.

How a Physical Therapist Is Different than a Chiropractor

Physical therapy and chiropractic care are very different. A chiropractor's philosophy as I understand it—I haven't studied chiropractic—is that everything centers around the spine and the alignment of the spine, and that all disease and injuries are based upon what they call subluxations of spinal segments. So, their philosophy is really come in, adjust them, and send them on their way.

Just like every other professional, there are good ones and bad ones. Now, some chiropractors will give their patients some exercises and some will do some soft tissue massage. In general, though, the difference is that when you go to a chiropractor they might do some scans and exams on you so they can determine what is the best course of action within their skill set. The problem with that is I see some chiropractors tend to keep people repeatedly coming back, never really empowering patients to fully take care of themselves. It seems to create a reliance on their services and I have seen some bad cases come out of this reliance if those patients are not properly managed. Let me point out, I'm not talking about all chiropractors. Some are very good about helping their patients. They will treat them for a few visits and then send them on their way with exercises and instructions that can help them in the long run.

Physical therapists tend to look at the entire patient. We look at the entire body and watch how they move, watch what deficits or imbalances they have, and look at strength, flexibility, mobility. Then we try to put that together into a moving picture for the patient so they can understand that if, say, they are having difficulty walking, it's because they have tightness here or weakness there. We help them see the bigger picture and how to resolve problems in the long term.

Much of what physical therapists do is centered on a lot of patient education. Many of our visits are a combination of manual therapy, exercises to specifically address the findings in our evaluations and use some modalities as needed, such as ultrasound or electric stimulation, to help with pain. But physical therapy is all about restoration of movement and return of the patient's functional mobility. Therefore, our profession is based upon identifying impairments, correcting those impairments and limitations, then trying to normalize and get the patient back to the best, balanced state of health and wellness.

The Distinction between a Physical Therapist and a Personal Trainer

There are marked differences between a physical therapist and a personal trainer. A physical therapist is someone who evaluates the whole body. We tend to look for areas of the body that are imbalanced, whether it's flexibility on one side of the body and not the other or weaknesses on one side. Again, we are highly skilled at addressing muscle imbalances, impairments, and restoring the patient back to normal mobility.

A physical therapist understands that when you are injured, certain muscles get tight and certain muscles get weak, and it's a very predictable pattern. We tend to give people very specific exercises to do that addresses those issues. We may try and stretch the areas that are tight, strengthen the opposite area, and facilitate the muscles to work properly in order to get people back to a balanced level.

When a personal trainer comes in, their focus is to get someone healthy, stronger, and in better shape. Unfortunately, personal trainers are not taught proper evaluative techniques and don't have the education to evaluate someone like physical therapists. What we often find is that when people are injured when working with personal trainers, it's because they had a muscle imbalance in their body prior to starting to exercise and then were overloaded with exercises they were not prepared for physically. The problem is if you try to build strength when you're out of balance, you can end up injured.

For example, if you're driving your car with the front wheels out of alignment such that they want to pull to the right, typically what you do is you go to a technician to correct the alignment so your car can drive straight. However, many people figure, "I'm weak, so I need to go to CrossFit", or "I need to go to a personal trainer." This mentality is essentially the same as thinking that the key is to drive faster with the hopes that driving faster will correct the alignment. But when you do that, you wear the tires out faster, you may wear the axle out, and you may start breaking down further down the line. People who have muscle imbalances and muscle weaknesses in specific areas are often very susceptible to injury if they start a CrossFit program or working with a personal trainer who is not trained to recognize these issues.

Why Healthy People Go to Physical Therapists

One of the fastest growing areas of our profession is people who come in and want to get more flexible, they want to get their core musculature stronger, and they want to be able to walk farther.

Physical therapy is not just for the injured. When someone comes to us when they don't have a nagging issue to deal with, that falls under our Wellness category. For these people, what we do is basically the same kind of evaluation that we do for an injured patient because we want to locate their imbalances, tight areas and weak areas. For example, if you have weak hip muscles, this will put more stress on your lower back when you walk or you hike.

A lot of times the majority of people in this population now have very weak core muscles. When they try to do more activities, they end up exercising on a very weak base and then they can end up getting hurt. Even though people may not have back pain yet, we try to teach them where their imbalances are, like tight hip flexors, weak glutes, or a weak core, and then give them strategies to help correct these findings and get them back to better health. If you try to push through this a little bit more, you're putting more and more stress on your lower back and you're probably going to end up getting hurt.

What to Do if You Sit for More Than Six Hours a Day

I always teach my patients that the human body is very resilient in the sense that it always tries to get back to its healing state. There have been studies on human tissues showing that if you take a piece of human tissue and place a load on the tissue for a period of about 20 minutes, you will distort it much like the beams of an old house bend. This phenomenon in physics is called "creep".

Creep is a physical property of mechanical distortion of materials under a load. The human body reacts in the same way with prolonged sitting. The vertical load in sitting distorts the lower back disc tissue. If you remove that weight, the body will rebound because it has elasticity in the tissue. The problem is after about 20 minutes, the ratio of recovery time is about a two to one ratio. For example, the 20-minute load that you put on the tissue would theoretically take 40 minutes of unloaded position to be able to recover. If you take someone who sits at their desk for eight hours, they are putting a lot of abnormal stress on their spine which creates a lot of disc pressure. To reverse this prolonged load from sitting, it would take literally 16 hours in an unloaded position, like lying on your back, to undo the effect of all that sitting in just one day. There are many other negative effects of sitting such as effects on your cardiovascular and respiratory systems. We as human beings are not meant to sit still.

I always tell my patients that if we think back in terms of evolution and the days of the caveman, if we sat still what would happen? Either your food source would move away from you or you would be eaten. We need to move. We are born and genetically made to move. The problem now is that technology has created a world of convenience and sedentary lifestyles. This is negatively affecting our health and wellness and is placing greater stresses on our backs. Sitting is now considered the new smoking, where it causes more and more problems the more we sit.

I educate my patients that if you are someone who has to sit for long periods at work, set up your office to where you have to get up and move to do something. If you have to fax something, put it across the room so you have to get up and move to go fax it. Same thing with a copier. Make sure you're changing your environment all the time. If you are one who is on the phone, get a headset. Every time the phone rings, stand up and move while you talk.

There are activities that someone who is a desk jockey can do that are good for you. It all comes back to movement. You can do a little unloading exercise by placing your arms on the armrest of the chair, lift yourself up out of the chair by extending your elbows to be fully straight and let your butt kind of hang from the spine. This unloads the spine by reversing the compression caused by sitting. There are many activities that someone who sits a lot can do. It's a matter of do they WANT to do it, and do they WANT to prevent the injury or a potential injury from happening?

The Common Mistake People Make When Working Toward Better Health and Wellness

A common mistake I often see after someone hears about the "Checks and Balances" concept is thinking that this concept is too simple and will not work. I challenge you to try it. Your progress must start here. This is not just another self-help book, or 'fix-it' book. I provide a simple, workable solution to help overcome back pain, stress, or whatever is affecting your life.

The second biggest mistake is not truly committing yourself to making a change. No commitment is the same as doing nothing. Your successes will never outpace the amount of effort you put into personal development and growth. We are often derailed by fears. Fears can hold us back from progressing forward. My coach once told me a valuable phrase, "Action cures fear. Procrastination and indecision fertilize fear."

The third mistake I see is trying to do this alone. Many people want to try to make improvements and keep the results to themselves but you are more likely to fail because we tend to quit easily at the first sign of failure or lack of progress. Find a friend, co-worker, neighbor or spouse, anyone to make the changes with you or go through the process together. There is nothing like holding yourself accountable to another person to make you follow through.

The fourth mistake is not being totally honest and truthful about where you are right now. Many of us don't like to face the reality of our current situation. We justify or rationalize why we are in the state we are in. For example, we use excuses and rationalizations to protect ourselves from failing. I hear many back pain patients say, "I couldn't get to my exercises because I was busy." To me, that means they are not serious about their condition. When they are not serious, they will not attend to themselves. When they are called to the table and held accountable, they will give every other reason to justify why they didn't do something instead of being totally honest and saying, "I know, I was not fully committed to it yesterday, but going forward, I will do my exercises every day." The proof is in the pudding. If someone wants to get better, then they really have to WANT to get better.

The Myths in the Wellness Industry

There are several myths in the physical therapy, health and wellness industry and the realm of self-improvement that need to be exposed and clarified.

1. "Physical therapy is basically getting a massage and ultrasound."

I get this at least once a day, if not more. Physical therapy is about movement and functional restoration. We are trained in anatomy, physiology, exercise physiology, and movement analysis. When you combine all of our education and experience, we are the ONLY healthcare providers who can help people get their function back. Soft tissue mobilization may be part of the equation to getting better, but NO ONE has ever improved his or her life for the long term with a 45-60 minute massage and a 10 minute ultrasound. People need to realize that if a person comes in for a massage with a complaint of tight muscles, the massage will help to loosen up those muscles but if the posture is not corrected and the activities that are contributing to creating those tight muscles, the muscles will ALWAYS return to the state that they were in before the massage.

Also, it is important to realize that what ultrasound does is to improve local circulation and the effects of ultrasound only lasts approximately 2-3 hours. Therefore, the benefits of massage and ultrasound are only temporary BUT combining soft tissue mobilization, stretching, mobilization and corrective exercises will help to create a long-lasting correction.

It is important to identify a person's impairments, limitations, and restrictions to create the right plan for them and to help get them back to the lifestyle they want to achieve. A physical therapy evaluation addresses all of these areas for every patient and will set the stage for a successful course of treatment.

2. "All physical therapy is the same."

Yes, we all share the same title, but it frustrates me when I hear about people who have been to physical therapy before and all they received was a hot pack, some ultrasound, a quick massage, and then sent home with some generic exercises. A quality physical therapist starts with an evaluation. During that evaluation, a good physical therapist listens to what the patient needs to determine what exactly is going on and what the patient needs to get back to what they want to do. Not all conditions are the same and not all conditions are treated the same. Just because your neighbor had back pain and took a pill that magically made the pain go away does not mean you will have the same result. For example, if someone comes in with a diagnosis of degenerative disc disease of the lumbar spine or stenosis of the lumbar spine, each patient may have other contributing factors that are unique to that patient. For example, one patient might also have a hip replacement, another might have diabetes, and another might have a past ankle fracture that is affecting their gait. Each of these conditions can affect the back in different ways and each patient needs to be individually evaluated to get to the correct course of action.

3. "Well, my dad has lower back pain (or whatever), so I knew I would get it."

Just because someone in your family had a condition or was suffering from some other issue, does that mean you are definitely heading in that direction? No. If your father had back pain, it may have been related to a job that he had as a laborer and he used poor body mechanics on the job. If you tend to sit at your desk all day, the stresses you place on your back are different than what your father did to his back and thus it really does not relate.

4. "I do exercises for my back - I do sit ups."

Sit-ups are probably the WORST exercise you can do for your back. It has been shown that doing typical sit-ups increases the pressure within the lumbar discs significantly greater than other exercises like static planks. We all need to keep our core musculature strong, but we want to do it with exercises that mimic our activities in life. For example, we want to develop our abdominals to stabilize our spines and protect our spines during movement. Therefore, we do stabilization exercises where we cue our patients to maintain their spinal position using the abdominals while superimposing arm and leg movements. Doing sit-ups does not replicate any activity that we do on a daily basis. They are useless! Bottom line, sit-ups or crunches are NOT core exercises.

5. "I do yoga. That is all I need."

Yoga is extremely beneficial. Don't get me wrong. Yoga is wonderful for stress reduction and flexibility. However, it is not a one-stop shop. I use an analogy in my practice of thinking about health and activity like a salad bar. Imagine a salad bar that is expansive and has lots of different choices of lettuces, toppings, dressing, etc. This is how we all should approach health and wellness. If you went to the same salad bar each day and had the same two or three items, you are getting some nutrients and essential vitamins from that salad, but there are so many more activities to try that have amazing potentials to improve your health. Going back to the salad bar and committing yourself to trying something new every time will add variety and keep you healthy.

6. "It is just the way it is, I can't change that."

Wrong, wrong, wrong! We have the power and choice to change anything we want to change. The operative word in that last sentence is WANT. You must have the desire to change and to WANT it, not need it, in order to make improvements. The one truth is that nothing in this world stays the same. Either everything gets better or worse, it never stays the same. As Henry Ford once said, "Whether you think you can or think you can't, you're right." If you feel that you can't change your back pain, well then, you can't. However, I know from 20 years of experience that you can improve back pain and learn to manage it successfully and actually prevent it from coming back!

7. "I don't have time to deal with this."

The question is, do you have time to live with all of the negative activities going on? What would happen if you did not do anything about a work situation? Your weight? Your back pain? Will they spontaneously get better or will they gradually get worse? Answer: the latter.

My experience with this question is do you have not only the time, but the patience and money to deal with a back problem that could take you out of work, possibly result in surgery and potential disability? If we put a little time and effort into our health every day, it pays dividends in return for many years to come. The saying I love is "an apple a day keeps the doctor away." We can manipulate this saying a bit in relation to our backs. How about, "a plank a day, keeps the physical therapist and spine surgeon away!"

How to Easily Achieve Optimal Health and Wellness

If you find yourself with pain of any kind, you can call our office and speak to someone on our team. We have two locations. Our Novato location phone number is 415-898-1311. Our San Anselmo location phone number is 415-457-4454. If you call in, our front desk team can get you started and get you on the right direction.

If you want to email us, you can email us at info@sstmarin.com. That will come directly into my office manager's mailbox. If you have a question for a physical therapist that will be forwarded to a physical therapist and one of our therapists will get back to you as soon as possible. It can be forwarded to me, which often happens, and I can answer questions first hand.

You can call one of our offices and ask to set up an appointment. We offer 15-minute FREE consultations for people who are not sure about what we do and want to ask some questions. Again, these consultations are free.

There are many different options for coming in and seeing us and knowing what to do for the next step – but the first step is to take action for yourself and to call our office.

I encourage anyone and everyone who is looking for a change to contact us. If you are local to our office, call us today to set up an appointment to help improve whatever pains you are experiencing. We offer full evaluations and treatment plans for those who are ready to commit to getting better and free consultations for those who want to find out more.

Even if you are not local to our office, you may give us a call and we can help get you started on your path to better health, fitness, and well-being. For many, we can help you navigate how to find a quality physical therapist in your neighborhood.

For those who are serious about improving and want to achieve exponential growth in life, health, business, and wellness, contact me to enroll in our coaching programs. Our Exponential Achievement Coaching programs will help you to get on track for the most amazing successes in your life, business, health, and wellness.

**Here's How to Easily Achieve
Optimal Health and Wellness**

You already know how debilitating even a little bit of pain is. Ninety percent of the population will end up with lower back pain that will last 6-8 weeks at minimum causing them to miss work and social events.

The confusing part is not knowing how to get back to feeling great after an injury, without getting bogged down in the quick to dole out medication to mask the pain healthcare system.

That's where we come in. We help people like you achieve optimal health and wellness while addressing the real cause of the pain.

Step 1: Call our Novato office at is 415-898-1311 or our San Anselmo office at 415-457-4454 to schedule a free, 15 minute Free Consultation or get started with a Physical Therapy evaluation right away.

Step 2: During the Free Consultation we determine your existing level of function, your health and wellness goals and determine what the next best step is for you with the programs that we offer. If you choose to get started right away in physical therapy, then the evaluation will help to identify the areas where you can improve and a comprehensive treatment plan will be designed for you with your goals in mind.

Step 3: After setting up the appointment, we take it from there and design an individualized evaluation and treatment plan aimed at getting you to optimal health quickly.

Most people think the solution to their aches and pains is to medicate it away, wait it out or just ignore it.

Now you can get the relief you need from the pain, but also get to the root cause of your injury so it doesn't happen again.

If you'd like us to help, just send an email to: info@sstmarin.com and we will take it from there.